A guide to establishing a national haemovigilance system

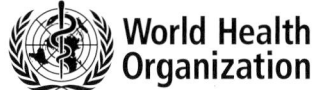
World Health Organization

WHO Library Cataloguing-in-Publication Data

A guide to establishing a national haemovigilance system.

I.World Health Organization.

ISBN 978 92 4 154984 4
Subject headings are available from WHO institutional repository

© World Health Organization 2016

All rights reserved. Publications of the World Health Organization are available on the WHO website (http://www.who.int) or can be purchased from WHO Press, World Health Organization, 20 Avenue Appia, 1211 Geneva 27, Switzerland (tel.: +41 22 791 3264; fax: +41 22 791 4857; email: bookorders@who.int).

Requests for permission to reproduce or translate WHO publications –whether for sale or for non-commercial distribution– should be addressed to WHO Press through the WHO website (http://www.who.int/about/licensing/copyright_form/index.html).

The designations employed and the presentation of the material in this publication do not imply the expression of any opinion whatsoever on the part of the World Health Organization concerning the legal status of any country, territory, city or area or of its authorities, or concerning the delimitation of its frontiers or boundaries. Dotted and dashed lines on maps represent approximate border lines for which there may not yet be full agreement.

The mention of specific companies or of certain manufacturers' products does not imply that they are endorsed or recommended by the World Health Organization in preference to others of a similar nature that are not mentioned. Errors and omissions excepted, the names of proprietary products are distinguished by initial capital letters.

All reasonable precautions have been taken by the World Health Organization to verify the information contained in this publication. However, the published material is being distributed without warranty of any kind, either expressed or implied. The responsibility for the interpretation and use of the material lies with the reader. In no event shall the World Health Organization be liable for damages arising from its use.

Printed in France.

Contents

Preface	**1**
Acknowledgements	**2**
1. Introduction	**3**
1.1 Goal of haemovigilance	3
1.2 Benefits of haemovigilance	3
1.3 Characteristics of successful haemovigilance systems	5
2. Organizational models for a national haemovigilance system	**6**
3. Prerequisites for an effective national haemovigilance system	**9**
3.1 Policy and legislative framework	9
3.2 Leadership and governance	10
3.3 Quality systems	10
3.4 Organization and coordination	10
3.5 Human and financial resources	10
3.6 Traceability	11
4. Planning a national haemovigilance system	**12**
5. Organization and coordination of haemovigilance activities	**14**
5.1 Haemovigilance in the donation and provision of blood and blood products	15
5.2 Haemovigilance in clinical transfusion	15
5.3 National haemovigilance activity	16
6. National management and use of haemovigilance data	**18**
6.1 Standard forms	18
6.2 Analysis and feedback reporting	19
6.3 Rapid alert systems	20
7. Capacity and skill building in haemovigilance	**21**
8. Monitoring, evaluation and outcomes	**23**
9. International haemovigilance activity	**24**
Glossary	**25**

Annexes   **26**

1. Standardized template form for the notification of a complication or an adverse reaction in a donor by the blood establishment   28

2. Standardized template form for the notification of an adverse event in a blood establishment: part A, rapid notification   30

3. Standardized template form for the notification of an adverse event in a blood establishment: part B, confirmation and finalization   31

4. Standardized template form for the notification of an adverse reaction in a recipient: part A, rapid notification by the hospital   32

5. Standardized template form for the notification of an adverse reaction in a recipient: part B, confirmation and finalization of the notification by the hospital   34

6. Standardized template form for the notification of an adverse event in a hospital: part A, rapid notification   35

7. Standardized template form for the notification of an adverse event in a hospital: part B, confirmation and finalization of a notification   36

8. Standardized periodic reporting template on complications or adverse reactions observed in donors by blood establishments   37

9. Standardized periodic reporting template on adverse events occurring in blood establishments   39

10. Standardized annual reporting template on adverse reactions observed in recipients by hospitals (health care institutions)   41

11. Standardized annual reporting template on adverse events occurring in hospitals (health care institutions)   43

Preface

The World Health Organization Blood Transfusion Safety programme was established to develop strategies for blood safety and promote them on a global, regional and national basis through advocacy and the provision of technical support to WHO Member States.

WHO recognizes the importance of haemovigilance to identify and prevent occurrence or recurrence of transfusion-related unwanted events, and to increase the safety, efficacy and efficiency of blood transfusion, covering all activities of the transfusion chain from donor to recipient. Whilst national haemovigilance systems are well established in many countries, there is a lack of effective haemovigilance in many resource-limited settings, and implementation in such settings remains an important and challenging problem.

The primary aim of this document is to support countries where haemovigilance is not already in place in establishing effective national systems for haemovigilance throughout the transfusion chain.

The specific objectives are to provide:
- policy guidance on establishing a haemovigilance system as part of the national blood and health systems;
- information and technical guidance on the specific measures and actions needed to implement a haemovigilance system.

Other countries may find the document helpful in strengthening their existing systems.

The intended audience includes the following organizations and institutions:
- ministries of health;
- bodies responsible for policy-making on blood safety, such as national blood commissions or councils;
- regulatory agencies;
- public health institutions;
- blood transfusion services, blood centres and plasma collection centres;
- hospitals, including hospital blood banks or health care facilities where transfusion takes place;
- blood donor organizations and other nongovernmental organizations involved in blood donor education and recruitment;
- patient groups;
- scientific and professional bodies;
- developmental partners and international organizations.

Acknowledgements

The Blood Transfusion Safety programme in the WHO Department of Service Delivery and Safety wishes to express its thanks to the following experts in haemovigilance who contributed to the development of the guidance: Yasmin Ayob (National Blood Centre, Ministry of Health, Malaysia), Keorapetse Thelma Moleli (South African National Blood Service, South Africa), Jean-Claude Faber (International Haemovigilance Network (IHN), Matthew Kuehnert (Centers for Disease Control and Prevention (CDC), United States of America), Dorothy Stainsby (independent consultant, United Kingdom), Jo Wiersum (ISBT Working Party on Haemovigilance, TRIP Landelijk Hemovigilantie Bureau, the Netherlands), and Erica Wood (Transfusion Research Unit, Monash University, Australia). Special thanks are due to Paul Ashford (independent consultant, United Kingdom) for synthesizing the drafted chapters and preparing the final manuscript.

Critical reviews were provided by Justina Kordai Ansah (National Blood Services, Ghana), Soyong Kwon (National Red Cross Nambu Blood Centre, the Republic of Korea), Che Kit Lin (independent consultant, Hong Kong SAR, China), Geni Neumann de Lima Camara (independent consultant, Brazil), May Yassin Raouf (Sharjah Blood Transfusion and Research Centre, United Arab Emirates), and Ponlapat Rojnuckarin (Faculty of Medicine, Chulalongkorn University, King Chulalongkorn Memorial Hospital, Thailand).

The following WHO staff members contributed to the development and reviews of the document: Noryati Abu Amin, Junping Yu, Neelam Dhingra, Micha Nuebling, Hernan Montenegro (WHO headquarters), Yetmgeta Abdella (WHO Regional Office for the Eastern Mediterranean), André Loua (WHO Regional Office for Africa), and María Dolores Pérez-Rosales (WHO Regional Office for the Americas).

Development of this publication was supported by Cooperative Agreement Number GH001180 from the United States Centers for Disease Control and Prevention (CDC). Its contents are solely the responsibility of the authors and do not necessarily represent the official view of CDC.

1. Introduction

The transfusion of blood and blood products is a life-saving intervention. However, there are risks of adverse events associated with the donation of blood and its components, and with the transfusion of blood and blood products to patients. Adverse events include all reactions, incidents, near misses, errors, deviations from standard operating procedures and accidents associated with blood donation and transfusion. Learning from adverse events and identifying system problems can drive the introduction of measures to enhance the quality, safety, efficacy and cost-effectiveness of blood and blood products as well as of the donation and transfusion processes.

> **What is haemovigilance?**
>
> Haemovigilance is a set of surveillance procedures covering the entire transfusion chain, from the donation and processing of blood and its components, to their provision and transfusion to patients and their follow-up. It includes the monitoring, reporting, investigation and analysis of adverse events related to the donation, processing and transfusion of blood, and taking actions to prevent their occurrence or recurrence.

Haemovigilance was established in the mid-1990s in response to concerns regarding transfusion-transmitted viral infections. Since then, haemovigilance programmes have drawn attention to the importance of many previously unrecognized and potentially preventable adverse events, including incorrect blood component transfused, transfusion-related acute lung injury and bacterial contamination of platelets. The resulting modifications to transfusion policies, standards and guidelines, and improvements to processes in blood services and transfusion practices in hospitals, have led to improved patient safety.

More recently the scope of haemovigilance has been expanded to include adverse events in blood donors, thus helping to improve safety for the donor as well as the patient.

Haemovigilance should be fully integrated into the quality systems of all institutions involved with the blood and blood products supply chain, including donation, testing, processing, inventory management, storage and distribution, and clinical transfusion, to ensure donor and patient safety at all levels.

1.1 GOAL OF HAEMOVIGILANCE

The goal of haemovigilance is continuous quality improvement of the transfusion chain through corrective and preventive actions to improve donor and patient safety, improve transfusion appropriateness, and reduce wastage. At its core, a haemovigilance system resembles any continuous quality improvement cycle and shows the same elements and activities. As such, haemovigilance should be embedded into every step of the transfusion chain, and into every organization that has responsibility for a part of that chain.

1.2 BENEFITS OF HAEMOVIGILANCE

Table 1 shows ways in which haemovigilance can have a positive impact on many stakeholders throughout the blood transfusion chain.

Table 1. Benefits of haemovigilance

Stakeholder	Impact/outcome
Blood donor	■ improved donor safety with a reduction in the frequency and severity of donor complications
	■ greater confidence in the blood donation process
Blood transfusion service	■ improved donor retention and return
	■ early detection of deficiencies and weaknesses
	■ continuous improvement in the quality of the services and products
	■ improved public confidence and trust in the blood transfusion service system
Hospital blood bank and health care facility	■ reduction in errors, omissions and system failures
	■ systematic and consistent reporting of all adverse events
	■ development of skills and expertise in the area of total quality management
	■ reduction in adverse events
	■ better health care outcomes
	■ less medico-legal action with an overall improvement of the community's regard of a particular facility
Patients receiving transfusion therapy	■ reduced risk of harm due to adverse events
	■ greater confidence in the blood transfusion process
Physicians and other health care professionals	■ identification and mitigation of transfusion-associated risks
	■ identification and quantification of unavoidable complications
	■ feedback leading to improved practice
Regional and national health authorities, regulatory and health agencies	■ early detection of emerging pathogens and the implementation of measures to mitigate the associated risks
	■ identification and mitigation of non-infective risks
	■ identification of trends in adverse events and opportunity for timely corrective action
Community	■ better care and stewardship of the gift of blood donation
	■ improved donor and patient confidence and trust in the blood system

| International bodies, societies, organizations | ■ benchmarking, developing best practice and creating awareness |

Haemovigilance systems can improve donor and patient safety by:
- identifying trends in adverse events and reactions;
- determining root causes and raising awareness;
- providing evidence for the development and amendment of policies to improve practices;
- guiding research;
- functioning as a rapid alert and early warning of emerging risks;
- achieving and demonstrating improvement.

1.3 CHARACTERISTICS OF SUCCESSFUL HAEMOVIGILANCE SYSTEMS

Although national haemovigilance systems vary among countries, those that have been most successful demonstrate some common characteristics.

From an organizational perspective:
- an efficient, adequately resourced and sustainable national system, involving all relevant stakeholders;
- non-punitive environment and based on a learning culture;
- confidentiality (the source of submitted data being protected);
- an integral part of the quality system of health care establishments, encompassing the entire transfusion chain;
- traceability from the blood donor and blood unit to recipient and vice versa, allowing adverse events to be tracked and investigated, and corrective action to be implemented;
- standards and definitions in line with international recommendations;
- education and training;
- feedback reporting to the stakeholder community.

From an operational perspective:
- simple to use;
- clear and standardized reporting forms;
- written standard procedures to initiate, investigate and coordinate reports;
- timely reporting of trends with expert analysis and recommendations for improvement to minimize rates of occurrence or recurrence;
- mechanisms to monitor the implementation of corrective and preventive actions in a timely manner and to demonstrate improved safety and clinical outcomes.

2. Organizational models for a national haemovigilance system

There are a number of possible ways in which a national haemovigilance system can be organized. For a particular country the best model will depend on the way in which the blood and health systems are structured and administered, and will be influenced by social and cultural norms. Table 2 shows the spectrum of choices, but in practice a system may lie anywhere along the spectrum.

Table 2. Organizational models of national haemovigilance systems

Model	Explanation of options
Centralized vs decentralized	■ In a centralized model, there is a central haemovigilance office that receives reports from institutions responsible for managing the adverse event. Feedback reporting is via national reports available to all health care organizations. Clinical improvements are recommended at the national level and rolled out across all organizations. ■ In a decentralized model there is no central collation of information. There may be some collation at a lower level (e.g. state). Clinical improvements are identified and implemented locally.
Stand-alone vs linked	■ A stand-alone model would be a system operated by a body that is managerially independent of the service provider (e.g. a scientific or professional body). ■ Linked systems may be operated by blood transfusion services or other health care agencies. In such models it is essential to ensure managerial separation between haemovigilance and operational management to avoid conflict of interest.
Active surveillance vs passive surveillance	■ Active surveillance is based on proactive and targeted search for adverse events in a systematic way. ■ Passive surveillance is characterized by reporting of adverse events as they are recognized in a spontaneous way, allowing for actions based on a retrospective approach. ■ A system may combine elements of both active and passive surveillance.

Model	Explanation of options
Voluntary vs mandatory reporting	■ A voluntary model of reporting encourages but does not enforce reporting. It is dependent on the willingness of the clinicians and health care professionals to report adverse events. ■ A mandatory model is a statutory requirement that must be fulfilled by all health care workers and relevant stakeholders. ■ Systems may combine both mandatory and voluntary elements, for example where there is a mandatory requirement to notify events leading to death or major morbidity, but not less serious events.
Non-punitive vs punitive systems	■ In a non-punitive system, individuals are not punished for appropriately reporting adverse events and safety concerns. Information in the haemovigilance system is protected from use in the disciplinary process. ■ In a punitive system individuals may be punished for appropriately reporting adverse events or safety concerns. Such systems may discourage participation by instilling fear.
Anonymized vs identified	■ In an anonymized system the identities of the individuals or institutions involved in the adverse event may be reported into the haemovigilance system but are not identified in feedback reports. ■ In an identified system the identity of the individuals or institutions involved in the adverse event may be identified in feedback reports.
Comprehensive vs limited	■ A comprehensive system may request reporting of all types of adverse events and all levels of severity. ■ A system may be limited to a subset of adverse events; for example, the system may only require serious adverse events to be reported at national level.

It is recommended that a non-punitive and anonymized approach be used. Establishing such a system encourages individuals and organizations to report adverse events and to learn from them.

Furthermore, it is important that all health care workers involved in the transfusion chain understand that the objective of the system is to improve donor and patient safety and existing practices. They should be reassured, comfortable and not afraid to report incidents because they might be blamed for the occurrence.

The basic premise of a national haemovigilance system is the development of a coordinated approach to the continuous improvement of the safety, availability and appropriate use of blood and blood products and related activities across all organizations involved in the transfusion chain.

Regardless of the model used in a country, it is very important that the reporting process is simple and quick. Complex or time-consuming procedures will be burdensome and will result in poor participation. It is also essential that donor and patient confidentiality is maintained and to this end donor- or patient-identifiable information should not be recorded in haemovigilance reports.

Vigilance in the wider context

Vigilance has a broader role, beyond that of blood and blood products, in the public health and health care service of a country. Blood is a medical product of human origin. Biovigilance extends the term haemovigilance beyond blood to incorporate monitoring of adverse events associated with other medical products of human origin, such as tissue, organs, and cells used for transplantation. In addition, surveillance for adverse events associated with medications is referred to as pharmacovigilance. The scheme encompassing haemovigilance, biovigilance, pharmacovigilance and other health care-associated vigilance programmes may differ depending on the structure of public health and health care delivery in the country. There may be overlap between biovigilance and pharmacovigilance. For instance, plasma products are sometimes included in either haemovigilance or pharmacovigilance.

Where pharmacovigilance systems, patient safety agencies, or offices for health care standards are active within the same jurisdiction, haemovigilance systems should interact with these agencies for the purposes of leveraging efficiencies of operation.

3. Prerequisites for an effective national haemovigilance system

In order for a national haemovigilance system to be effective there needs to be a certain degree of national coordination of blood transfusion activity. Ideally the following should be in place:
- national blood policy and plan;
- legislative and regulatory framework;
- national blood commission or authority;
- well organized, nationally coordinated blood transfusion service;
- quality systems in blood transfusion services and hospitals (particularly their blood banks);
- hospital-based transfusion committees with oversight of all aspects of clinical transfusion practice.

WHO aide-mémoires on "National haemovigilance system", "National blood system", "Good policy process for blood safety and availability" and "The clinical use of blood" provide checklists to help in assessing the country situation.

In addition to these organizational aspects it is essential that the identification of blood products and the record keeping at each stage of the transfusion chain support bidirectional traceability (tracking from donor to recipient and vice versa).

3.1 POLICY AND LEGISLATIVE FRAMEWORK

At the highest level, the role of haemovigilance as an essential element of the safe blood donation and transfusion process should be recognized in the national blood policy. The fundamental structure or model of the haemovigilance system should be defined taking into account the structure of the national blood system and the health system. The options discussed in Section 2 above will need to be considered.

The haemovigilance element of the blood policy, and legislative and regulatory framework, should be developed in a manner that support stepwise implementation of haemovigilance, commencing at institutional level in accordance with the national structure or model and progressing to a nationally coordinated haemovigilance system.

The policy and legislative framework should:
- define the scope and nature of the haemovigilance system with the objective of national coordination;
- identify the organizational arrangements and the institution responsible for centrally coordinated haemovigilance;
- ensure adequate funding and human resources;
- define the respective roles and responsibilities of the different stakeholders;
- describe reporting and feedback mechanisms;
- specify monitoring and evaluation requirements.

3.2 LEADERSHIP AND GOVERNANCE

The ministry of health has ultimate responsibility for the national blood system and for the quality, safety and sufficiency of the supply of blood and blood products. The haemovigilance system contributes to the safety of donation, blood products and transfusion. It improves risk management, increases trust and should be confidential and non-punitive in nature. The ministry of health should provide effective leadership and governance for a national haemovigilance system and should define the scope and elements of the haemovigilance system.

3.3 QUALITY SYSTEMS

Within each organization that is responsible for elements of the transfusion chain an effective quality (management) system should be in place. This system should ensure consistent practice through the use of written procedures and regular audit. A quality improvement cycle should be in place producing demonstrable results through quality indicators.

In blood transfusion services there should be a comprehensive quality system in place and haemovigilance should be embedded within this system.

In hospitals, transfusion committees should be in place to ensure appropriate clinical use of blood, effective training of staff, and monitoring and evaluation of clinical practice. The transfusion committee should oversee the implementation of haemovigilance in the hospital, regularly review the results and monitor the effectiveness of improvement measures.

3.4 ORGANIZATION AND COORDINATION

Stakeholders and responsible organizations and institutions need to be identified. Roles and responsibilities need to be defined and appropriate coordination put in place. The ministry of health should:

- establish organizational arrangements and mechanisms to engage and coordinate all key stakeholders;
- define the roles, responsibilities and accountabilities of all stakeholders;
- facilitate international cooperation with existing haemovigilance networks.

3.5 HUMAN AND FINANCIAL RESOURCES

There needs to be recognition of the requirement for adequate human and financial resources for the establishment, development and sustainability of the haemovigilance system. Haemovigilance activities are required at every point in the transfusion chain.

As a priority, resources will need to be identified to support national coordination and to allow each organization involved in the transfusion chain to assign a nominated lead individual, ensure adequate training of staff, and provide the necessary equipment and time for staff to perform haemovigilance activities.

It is recommended that expertise in data collection, storage and analysis is recruited early in the process of planning a haemovigilance programme. Decisions on internal or outsourced capacity for data analysis need to be considered as part of project planning.

3.6 TRACEABILITY

Traceability describes the ability to reliably follow the information trail from donor to recipient and vice versa in a timely manner. Traceability is essential to ensure the ability to recall at-risk products, to identify recipients of non-conforming products that may require additional follow-up, and to fully investigate adverse events.

The key elements of traceability are:
- a system to uniquely identify each donor, donation (together with its associated samples and blood components) and recipient;
- a system for record keeping throughout the transfusion pathway that captures the identifiers at each stage and maintains necessary linkages;
- documentation of the actual administration of blood components to the intended recipient or of their final disposal;
- secure methods for transcription of critical data to ensure accuracy;
- system for information storage capable of retaining traceability records for long periods (e.g. European Union directives require traceability for 30 years from time of donation and transfusion);
- procedures that assist staff in following the traceability path (e.g. standard operating procedures to support look-back activity).

4. Planning a national haemovigilance system

The manner in which a national haemovigilance system is planned, developed and implemented will depend on the country situation and the organizational structure or model adopted. In most cases it is likely to be appropriate to adopt a nationally coordinated stepwise approach.

At the start of the process, there needs to be general consensus as to the need, benefit and implementation of such a system. Such consensus should include a clear understanding of how the system is to be designed, implemented and maintained, with particular attention to the level of complexity at which the system will operate and what the main objectives will be. A haemovigilance system requires interaction and coordination between multiple stakeholders involved in the provision, transfusion, surveillance and regulation of blood and blood products. Organizational arrangements and mechanisms should be put in place to coordinate and engage all key stakeholders. Stakeholders may include blood transfusion services, hospital blood banks, hospital transfusion committees, clinical departments, professional bodies, public health institutions and regulatory agencies, as well as patients and blood donor groups. The respective roles, responsibilities and accountabilities of all stakeholders should be clearly defined. The decision as to what should be reported by whom and to whom should be considered carefully, with due regard to available resources and systems.

The need for national leadership and coordination is of paramount importance in order to ensure consistent implementation across the country. A lead individual or team should be designated by the ministry of health with responsibility for the national haemovigilance system. Activities may be delegated to an external body such as a professional association or national public health organization, provided there are no conflicts of interest. Nevertheless, the final and overall responsibility for the haemovigilance system needs to remain with the ministry of health. The planning activities should include:

- setting the goals and objectives;
- designing the national haemovigilance system;
- identifying all the constituent elements and resource requirements;
- identifying educational needs and appropriate resources;
- defining the implementation steps and timetable;
- identifying stakeholders and establishing links and communication with participating organizations and institutions;
- identifying mechanisms to provide leadership, professional support and expert advice;
- identifying training and outreach activities to build awareness of the value of haemovigilance and the importance of reporting among stakeholders.

In determining the scope of the system, the following should be considered.

Should the system:
- include all adverse reactions in patients or serious adverse reactions only?
- include all errors and near misses with and without clinical consequences?

- include adverse events in patients, donors or both?
- Include an expert review of all or some events?
- report back immediately on adverse events, thus enabling rapid corrective or preventive action, or report back analysed data retrospectively (e.g. trends reported on an annual basis and follow-up of corrective measures)?

5. Organization and coordination of haemovigilance activities

A well established national haemovigilance system is based on active participation (i.e. submission of reports or a nil report) by all blood transfusion services and hospitals where blood donation and transfusion takes place. Participation is encouraged by ease of reporting (e.g. online reporting, simple forms, availability of non-judgemental professional advice), confidence that the report will make a contribution to safety improvements, and assurance of confidentiality for patients, donors and staff.

Haemovigilance activity should be implemented in all institutions and facilities responsible for any element of the blood transfusion chain. These local systems need to be developed in line with the national framework.

Within these organizations staff should be trained in the concepts of haemovigilance and quality improvement and given specific roles and responsibilities with regard to vigilance and reporting. A culture of teamwork and quality improvement should be encouraged.

An individual should be identified in each organization as the "transfusion safety officer" with responsibility for internally coordinating haemovigilance activity. In smaller organizations this may be a part-time responsibility, but in larger organizations a full-time position may be necessary.

National coordination of training and standardization of forms, procedures and educational materials is encouraged, as this will be cost-effective and will help ensure a consistent approach to haemovigilance at the national level.

Nationally standardized definitions, procedures, forms and reports should be used. All relevant staff should be trained and documentation of training should be kept. Responsibilities with respect to haemovigilance should be documented in the relevant job descriptions.

Within a given organization, adverse events (including adverse reactions in donors and patients, incidents, accidents, errors, deviations, near misses) should be handled in accordance with the requirements of the established quality management system, including the execution of appropriate corrective and preventive actions.

At the institutional level policies, guidelines, protocols and standard operating procedures (blood transfusion safety and clinical) should be developed for all processes.

All organizations involved in the transfusion chain should submit an annual report of haemovigilance activity, including relevant denominator data, to the national lead for haemovigilance.

5.1 HAEMOVIGILANCE IN THE DONATION AND PROVISION OF BLOOD AND BLOOD PRODUCTS

Blood transfusion services should implement a haemovigilance system embedded in their quality system. A named member of senior staff should be given lead responsibility for establishing and managing the system. The haemovigilance system should address the detection, identification, documentation and reporting of adverse events, including the following:

- events occurring before, during and after the donation of blood or blood components;
- release of non-conforming products;
- significant deviations from protocols;
- errors and near misses;
- adverse reactions with blood products delivered by the blood transfusion service.

The system should ensure the thorough investigation and documentation of adverse events and should include root cause analysis and corrective and preventive actions as part of a continuing improvement cycle.

The blood transfusion service should maintain close links with the hospitals (hospital blood bank, transfusion safety officers, transfusion committee, treating clinicians) they serve, and the blood transfusion service should provide assistance to hospitals in the investigation of adverse events.

Networking between haemovigilance leads in blood transfusion services should be encouraged.

5.2 HAEMOVIGILANCE IN CLINICAL TRANSFUSION

Every hospital and health care facility responsible for the transfusion of blood products should have a transfusion committee in place. A named individual within the transfusion committee should be given lead responsibility for haemovigilance (this could be the transfusion safety officer of the hospital). This individual should act as a liaison between the transfusion committee and other vigilance and control systems in the hospital (e.g. infection control, risk management).

The haemovigilance system should address the detection, identification, documentation and reporting of adverse events occurring in the hospital, including the following:

- errors in the collection and testing of blood samples;
- errors in the identification of patients;
- inappropriate use of blood products (e.g. accidental overtransfusion);
- incorrect blood product transfused;
- significant deviations from protocols;
- near misses;
- adverse reactions associated with the transfusion of blood products.

The system should include root cause analysis and corrective and preventive actions as part of a continuing improvement cycle.

The transfusion committee should maintain close links with the blood transfusion service that provides the blood products, so that investigation of adverse events can be efficient and timely measures can be initiated to prevent transfusion of related blood products.

Data from haemovigilance should link to clinical audit programmes, so that recommendations arising from haemovigilance reports can be incorporated into standards and guidelines, and compliance assessed and improved.

Networking between transfusion safety officers in different organizations should be encouraged. In all cases it is important that the transfusion safety officer has the time and financial resources available to fulfil their responsibilities.

5.3   NATIONAL HAEMOVIGILANCE ACTIVITY

Within a national framework, the responsibilities of a national haemovigilance office include:
- putting in place mechanisms for data collection, validation and analysis, publication and dissemination of reports, development of recommendations and monitoring implementation;
- receiving adverse event reports from blood transfusion services and hospitals;
- reviewing reports to ensure the quality of reporting;
- identifying trends and investigating underlying causes;
- providing expert guidance to address root causes and improve safety;
- identifying improvements in the processes of the transfusion chain;
- improving education in haemovigilance;
- producing an annual national haemovigilance report;
- possible development of a rapid alert and early warning platform to communicate and share information;
- linkage interfacing with other relevant national systems, regional schemes and international activities;
- periodic review, monitoring and evaluation of the haemovigilance system.

This national activity could be managed directly through the ministry of health or via a third party such as a professional body. Various models exist, but professional leadership is essential.

Engagement with national and international experts and professional societies should be encouraged to ensure the best possible advice and quality improvement.

Figure 1. Flow of haemovigilance data

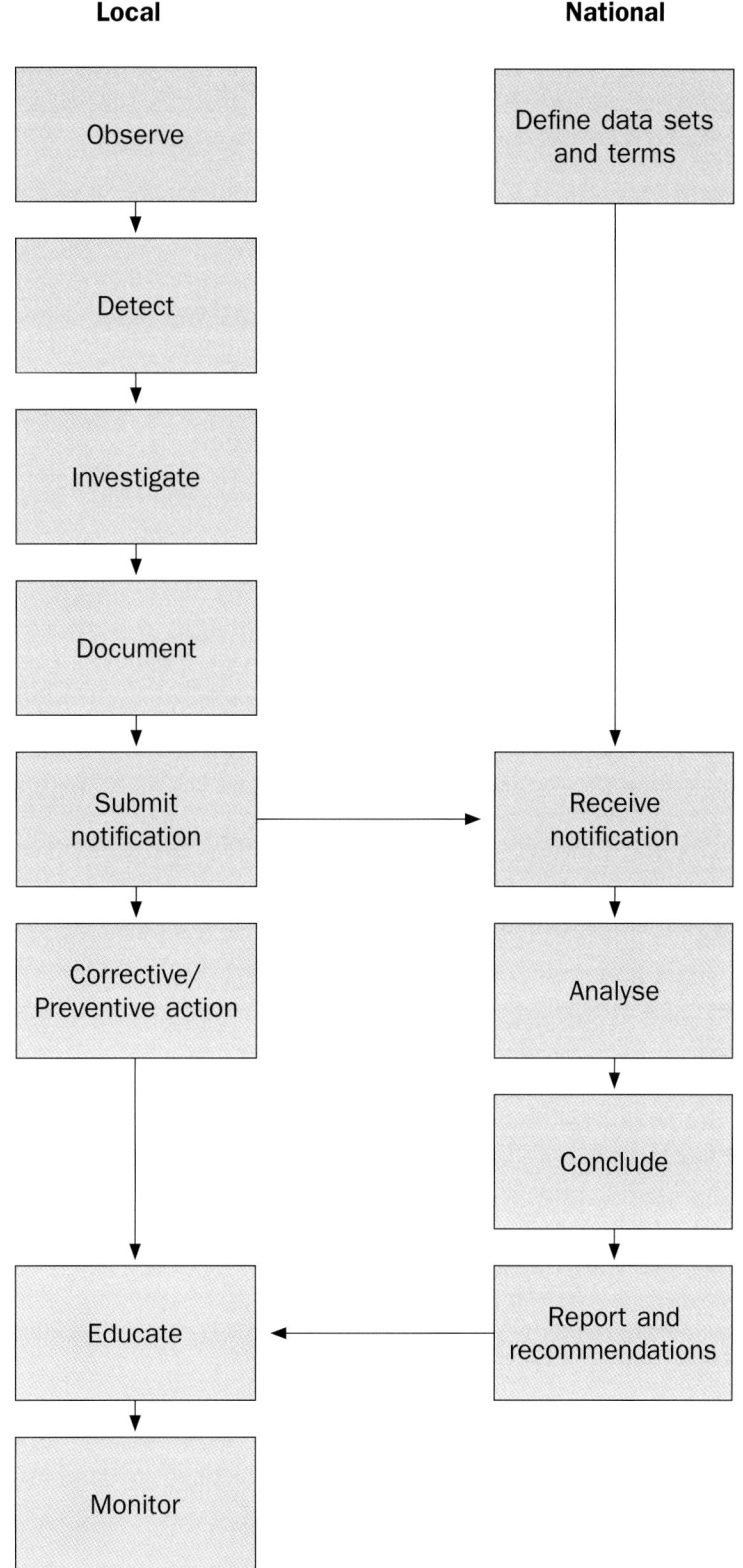

6. National management and use of haemovigilance data

Effective data collection and management is at the core of any successful national surveillance programme and requires clearly documented definitions, policies and procedures as well as defined roles and responsibilities.

As for any surveillance system, agreed definitions of adverse events and associated terms are crucial. These should be preferably aligned with international terminology to promote comparability of data collected across countries. International Society of Blood Transfusion (ISBT) and International Haemovigilance Network (IHN) standard definitions of adverse events, including severity and imputability levels, can be found at www.isbtweb.org and www.ihn-org.com, respectively.

A comprehensive data collection network should be established to ensure data can be collected from all blood transfusion services and sites where blood transfusion is undertaken. The type of information collected should be tailored to needs and capacity, and should preferably be scalable, to allow the scope and the level of detail to be extended as the system matures. The system design should describe who should report, to whom, and how this should be done. Sophisticated web-based systems may be the ideal; however, simple but accurate reporting and analysis of manually collected data may be as effective in bringing about sustained improvement in blood safety.

Effective traceability is fundamental. The type of system will depend on the availability of resources and the level of development of the blood system in the country.

A national haemovigilance data management system requires the following:
- confidentiality and anonymity for donors, patients and reporters;
- data security and compliance with applicable regulations on data protection;
- minimal impact of data collection on the working methods of the blood transfusion centre or health care system;
- expert and non-judgemental advice and guidance on investigation, management, reporting and follow-up of adverse events;
- expert analysis of events and trends and provision of clear recommendations for improvement.

The flow of haemovigilance data is illustrated in Figure 1, showing the relationship between local (including institutional) and national activity.

The rigorous and transparent management of information generated through this system has a key role in introducing amendments in blood policies and guidelines that lead to improvements in processes and practices in donation and transfusion.

6.1 STANDARD FORMS

Reporting should be performed using a standard form, either by a paper or electronic system. A two-stage method of adverse event reporting may be used, in which an initial short report is submitted, followed by a more detailed report when investigations are completed.

Adverse event reports to the national system should not include information that could identify the patient, donor, reporter or any other individual involved, but should include a unique identifier enabling the national haemovigilance coordinator to request further details if necessary.

The adverse event report should include:

- a description of the adverse event or near miss;
- a graded assessment of the clinical outcome (from no reaction or minor signs to death, i.e. the severity);
- an assessment of the probability that the adverse event was caused by the transfusion (i.e. the imputability);
- information on action taken by the blood centre or hospital.

Examples of generic forms can be found in the annexes. These can be used for guidance but should be adapted to the national situation.

Reports should be scrutinized to ensure that they are correctly categorized, and that all relevant information has been documented, such as results of laboratory investigations in the case of adverse reactions, or root cause analysis of errors. This may require dialogue between the national haemovigilance coordinator and the reporter.

In systems that collect both serious and less serious events, the expert review of submitted reports may be mainly focused on the serious events.

6.2 ANALYSIS AND FEEDBACK REPORTING

Haemovigilance data should be analysed centrally and an aggregate feedback report compiled and distributed to all organizations involved in the blood transfusion chain and other stakeholders. The feedback report should include recommendations for implementation of preventive action (this could be by hospitals, blood centres or ministries of health) and it should be issued in a timely manner, to ensure effective use of the data to improve practice and to encourage submission of data. The inclusion of illustrative anonymized case studies may be useful for educational and training purposes. Generic template reporting forms can be found in the annexes and these provide a resource to assist in designing the national feedback report.

When assessing the probability that an adverse event will occur it is necessary to know both the number of occasions on which the adverse event has occurred (the numerator data) and the number of times the associated procedure or process has occurred in total (the denominator data). For example, if a blood centre sends three reports of virus transmission in a year and the total volume of blood provided by that centre is 120 000 units, then the risk of transmission is 1 in 40 000. However, if the total volume of blood provided is 6000 units, the risk of transmission is 1 in 2000.

For patient (recipient) vigilance the ideal denominator is the number of units of the relevant blood product transfused and the number of patients receiving the blood product. However, accurate data on products transfused may not be available and in such cases a surrogate, such as the number of units of blood products distributed from the blood transfusion service to the hospital or issued from the hospital blood bank to the clinical area, can be used.

If available, demographic and clinical data on transfused patients (e.g. sex, age, disease or indication for transfusion) can help identify patients at higher risk of an adverse event.

For donor vigilance reports the denominator data may be the number of donations collected or the number of times potential donors present. Adverse events may thus be expressed as, for example, number per 100 000 whole blood donations. Where possible, both adverse reactions or complications and collections should be broken down into the main collection types: whole blood donation versus apheresis, first-time donors versus repeat donors.

Benchmarking and comparison of haemovigilance data between hospitals, blood transfusion centres and even countries requires reliable and correct denominator data.

6.3 RAPID ALERT SYSTEMS

The haemovigilance system may include a rapid alert or early warning mechanism for the rapid dissemination of information on important events, emerging hazards or trends. Such a system should not replace urgent notification to the blood centre of adverse events requiring immediate action, e.g. post-transfusion sepsis or blood bag defects.

7. Capacity and skill building in haemovigilance

Appropriate education, training and competency assessment of all health care personnel involved in blood transfusion activities are essential. All personnel involved in the blood transfusion chain, from the blood transfusion service, the hospital blood bank through to the clinical areas, should be trained in safe handling and administration of blood products and in haemovigilance. Training should include the general principles of haemovigilance, its objectives and benefits, and individual roles and responsibilities.

Skill building is a continuous process that includes:
- role-specific training for all staff involved in the transfusion chain and for management of donor and patient complications;
- availability of current standard operating procedures and practice guidelines;
- documentation of training;
- competency assessment.

Staff training, education and competence assessment are the responsibility of educational establishments, health authorities, hospitals and blood transfusion services.

The objective is that all health care personnel involved in blood transfusion are competent in safe practice, aware of the implications of errors and alert to adverse events, and also understand the importance of reporting to the haemovigilance system in order to contribute to safety and quality improvements. It should be explicit that the aim of the programme is to improve blood transfusion practice; it is not intended as a punitive exercise.

Examples of education and training activities include:
- pre-service training of doctors, nurses, laboratory scientists, pharmacists and other health care workers in:
  — appropriate prescribing;
  — safe bedside procedures, correct patient identification and pre-transfusion sampling and labelling;
  — safe administration of blood and blood products;
  — recognizing, investigating and managing adverse reactions and events in patients or donors;
  — practice of haemovigilance;
- in-service training in good working practices, including an understanding of quality systems and the need to follow standard operating procedures;
- haemovigilance-specific training that ensures a good understanding of:
  — the rationale and concept of haemovigilance;
  — the national haemovigilance programme;
  — detecting, recognizing, investigating and reporting adverse events;
  — conducting root cause analysis;
  — applying corrective and preventive actions to improve practice.

Regular competency assessment should be carried out and documented to ensure that staff retain the necessary skills and knowledge for their specific roles in the transfusion chain.

Staff with a lead or coordinating role in haemovigilance will require more specific training in how to establish, manage, maintain and monitor a haemovigilance system. Such individuals will require a broad knowledge of evidence-based transfusion practices and technical skills related to transfusion safety, together with leadership qualities, effective communication and teaching skills, and ability to influence practice and effect change.

National haemovigilance leads will need further skills, including:
- establishing and managing a central coordinating office;
- developing tools for data collection;
- characterizing adverse events;
- verifying reports;
- advising on investigation and root cause analysis of events;
- analysing and managing data;
- producing annual feedback reports and educational material;
- liaising with professional groups and stakeholder organizations.

Training at all levels should be regularly updated in response to haemovigilance reports and practice guidelines to ensure improvements to practice become embedded in the curriculum.

8. Monitoring, evaluation and outcomes

Monitoring and evaluation plays a critical role in ensuring that the system is functioning effectively and can adapt over time to changing circumstances and environments. A plan should be developed to monitor the development of the haemovigilance system and evaluate its impact on a regular basis. Regular evaluation also provides objective evidence in support of the programme's continuation and is crucial for its sustainability.

Haemovigilance systems, regardless of how successfully they have been implemented, all face certain limitations. Possible limitations and drawbacks include:
- low participation;
- incomplete reporting;
- missing details;
- variation in terminology and definitions;
- failure to detect transfusion association, particularly with events not detected until some time after the transfusion event (e.g. some infections);
- influence of the health care system's or institution's "culture" regarding compliance, process improvement and reporting.

Process and outcome indicators should be developed to track planned haemovigilance activities and assess the effective functioning and success of the haemovigilance system. When problems are detected in the haemovigilance system, these should be actively investigated and adequate measures taken to better serve the objectives of the system.

The impact of the haemovigilance system in contributing to changes in policies and practices in donation, processing and transfusion is dependent on its links to bodies with responsibility for policy and guideline development, for example:
- national and regional transfusion committees;
- professional bodies (medical, nursing, technical and scientific);
- blood transfusion services;
- hospitals and other health care facilities;
- ministry of health;
- regulatory agencies.

Evaluation of the haemovigilance system should therefore include an appraisal of the effectiveness of these links and the extent to which they are used to promote improvements in donation and transfusion safety.

9. International haemovigilance activity

Haemovigilance collaborations, such as the International Haemovigilance Network and the Working Party on Haemovigilance of the International Society of Blood Transfusion (ISBT), are initiatives that aim to stimulate country participation in global haemovigilance and develop and maintain worldwide common structures on blood safety and haemovigilance. Some of the main objectives of an international network are to encourage exchange of valuable information, initiate joint activities between the members, offer support and assistance to each other, provide specific educational activities, review and standardize definitions, organize meetings and consultations, and contribute to the running of an international haemovigilance database.

The International Surveillance of Transfusion-Associated Reactions and Events (ISTARE) is an international database on haemovigilance that collects aggregate data from participating haemovigilance systems and members of the International Haemovigilance Network (IHN).[1] It has a holistic approach, collecting data on recipients and donors and on all adverse events, not only serious ones. The data sets are anonymized and are only known to the respective participant.

ISTARE is now fully operational in web-based form. If you are the authorized person, you may enter, by following simple steps, your country's haemovigilance data. You may enter data for previous years as well as the most recent data. Your country will not be identified by name in ISTARE output; it can only be recognized by a code that will be known exclusively to you.

Wherever possible national schemes should make use of international standards, definitions and best practice.

The Notify Library[2] provides a reference platform where experts from across the globe collaborate to share didactic information on documented adverse outcomes associated with the application of substances of human origin, e.g. organs, blood, tissues and cells. The library aims to support continued improvements in safety and efficacy in transplantation, transfusion and assisted reproduction.

---

[1] www.ihn-org.com/haemovigilance-databases/istare-2.
[2] http://www.notifylibrary.org/.

Glossary

The glossary below reflects the usage of the terms in the current document.

Adverse event	Any undesirable or unintended occurrence associated with transfusion or donation. It includes all adverse reactions, incidents, near misses, errors, deviations from standard operating procedures and accidents.
Adverse event reporting	Sending information on adverse events to the haemovigilance system for further investigation, analysis and feedback.
Adverse reaction	Any unintended response in donor or patient associated with the collection or transfusion of blood or blood components.
Corrective action	Action taken to eliminate the cause of a detected nonconformity or other undesirable situation.
Haemovigilance feedback report	Report of aggregated analysed data from the haemovigilance system.
Imputability	The probability that an identified probable cause was the actual cause of an adverse event after the investigation of the adverse transfusion event is completed.
Incident	Any untoward occurrence associated with an activity or process, such as the collection, testing, processing, storage and distribution of blood and blood components, or in the transfusion or administration.
Near miss	An error or deviation from standard procedures or policies which, if undetected, could result in the determination of a wrong blood group or issue, collection or administration of an incorrect, inappropriate or unsuitable component, but which was recognized before the transfusion took place.
Notification	Mandatory information on a notifiable event to the regulatory authority.
Preventive action	Action taken to eliminate the cause of a potential nonconformity or other potential undesirable situation.

Annexes

The following annexes contain templates of forms for notification and reporting.

They are examples to facilitate start-up of a haemovigilance system and standardization of haemovigilance procedures, as they are based on existing templates, in line with internationally agreed definitions and terminologies.

They can and should be adapted to the local situation.

TEMPLATES OF FORMS FOR HAEMOVIGILANCE

1. Blood establishment

Notification of a complication or adverse reaction in a donor by the blood establishment

Annex 1. Standardized template form for the notification of a complication or an adverse reaction in a donor by the blood establishment (to be used for an individual incident by the blood establishment to inform the central haemovigilance unit)

Notification of an adverse event in a blood establishment: part A, rapid notification

Annex 2. Standardized template form for the notification of an adverse event in a blood establishment – rapid notification (to be used for an individual incident by the blood establishment to inform the central haemovigilance unit)

Notification of an adverse event in a blood establishment: part B, confirmation and finalization

Annex 3. Standardized template form for the notification of an adverse event in a blood establishment – confirmation and finalization notification (to be used for an individual incident by the blood establishment to inform the central haemovigilance unit)

2. Hospitals

Notification of an adverse reaction in a hospital: part A, rapid notification

Annex 4. Standardized template form for the notification of an adverse reaction in a recipient – rapid notification by the hospital (to be used for an individual incident by the hospital to inform the central haemovigilance unit)

Notification of an adverse reaction in a hospital: part B, confirmation and finalization

Annex 5. Standardized template form for the notification of an adverse reaction in a recipient – confirmation and finalization of the notification by the hospital (to be used for an individual incident by the hospital to inform the central haemovigilance unit)

Notification of an adverse event in a hospital: part A, rapid notification

Annex 6. Standardized template form for the notification of an adverse event in a hospital – rapid notification (to be used for an individual incident by the hospital to inform the central haemovigilance unit)

Notification of an adverse event in a hospital: part B, confirmation and finalization

Annex 7. Standardized template form for the notification of an adverse event in a hospital – confirmation and finalization of a notification (to be used for an individual incident by the hospital to inform the central haemovigilance unit)

TEMPLATES FOR REPORTING ON HAEMOVIGILANCE

Blood establishments

Periodic reporting template: complications or adverse reactions in blood establishments

Annex 8. Standardized periodic reporting template on complications or adverse reactions observed in donors by blood establishments (for internal and external purposes; for monthly, trimestrial, semestrial and annual reporting)

Periodic reporting template: adverse events in blood establishments

Annex 9. Standardized periodic reporting template on adverse events occurring in blood establishments (for internal and external purposes; for monthly, trimestrial, semestrial and annual reporting)

Hospitals

Annual reporting template: adverse reactions in hospitals

Annex 10. Standardized annual reporting template on adverse reactions observed in recipients by hospitals (health care institutions) (to be used for internal and external purposes, inter alia to inform the central haemovigilance unit)

Annual reporting template: adverse events in hospitals

Annex 11. Standardized annual reporting template on adverse events occurring in hospitals (health care institutions) (to be used for internal and external purposes, inter alia to inform the central haemovigilance unit)

Template form for haemovigilance in the blood establishment

ANNEX 1. STANDARDIZED TEMPLATE FORM FOR THE NOTIFICATION OF A COMPLICATION OR AN ADVERSE REACTION IN A DONOR BY THE BLOOD ESTABLISHMENT

(to be used for an individual incident by the blood establishment to inform the central haemovigilance unit)

Complication (adverse reaction) in a donor

Reporting blood establishment _____

Report identification _____

Date complication/adverse reaction occurred (*year/month/day*) _____

Date of notification (*year/month/day*) _____

Type of donation:
☐ Whole blood
☐ Platelets (apheresis)
☐ Plasma
    ☐ apheresis
    ☐ manual
☐ Combined (apheresis)
☐ Other (*specify*):

Type of donor complication or adverse reaction(s)	Severity level			
	1	2	3	4
Vasovagal				
Haematoma				
Damage to vessel (vein or artery)				
Damage to nerve				
Specific apheresis complication				
■ allergic reaction (generalized)				
■ anaphylaxis				
■ haemolysis				
■ embolism				
■ hypotension (induced due to hypovolemia)				
■ clotting				
■ citrate intoxication				
Other reaction(s) (*specify*):				

Remarks: _____

_____

Notified by: _____

to: _____

Date: _____

ANNEX 2. STANDARDIZED TEMPLATE FORM FOR THE NOTIFICATION OF AN ADVERSE EVENT IN A BLOOD ESTABLISHMENT: PART A, RAPID NOTIFICATION

(to be used for an individual incident by the blood establishment to inform the central haemovigilance unit)

Notification of an adverse event
Part A: <u>Rapid</u> notification of an adverse event

Reporting blood establishment _____

Report identification _____

Reporting date (*year/month/day*) _____

Date of adverse event (*year/month/day*) _____

Serious adverse event, which may affect quality and safety of blood component due to a deviation in:	Specification			
	Product defect	**Equipment failure**	**Human error**	**Other** (*specify*)
Whole blood collection				
Apheresis collection				
Testing of donations				
Processing				
Storage				
Distribution				
Materials				
Others (specify)				

Remarks: _____

Notified by: _____

to: _____

Date: _____

ANNEX 3. STANDARDIZED TEMPLATE FORM FOR THE NOTIFICATION OF AN ADVERSE EVENT IN A BLOOD ESTABLISHMENT: PART B, CONFIRMATION AND FINALIZATION

(to be used for an individual incident by the blood establishment to inform the central haemovigilance unit)

Notification of an adverse event

Part B: **Confirmation** and **finalization** of a notification of an adverse event in a blood establishment

Reporting establishment _____

Report identification _____

Confirmation date (*year/month/day*) _____

Date of serious adverse event (*year/month/day*) _____

Root cause analysis (*details*) _____

_____

_____

Corrective measures taken (*details*) _____

_____

_____

Template form for haemovigilance in the hospital

ANNEX 4. STANDARDIZED TEMPLATE FORM FOR THE NOTIFICATION OF AN ADVERSE REACTION IN A RECIPIENT: PART A, RAPID NOTIFICATION BY THE HOSPITAL

(to be used for an individual incident by the hospital to inform the central haemovigilance unit)

Notification of a serious adverse reaction

Part A: **Rapid** notification for a suspected adverse reaction in a recipient

Reporting establishment _____

Report identification _____

Reporting date (*year/month/day*) _____

Age and sex of recipient _____

Date of transfusion (*year/month/day*) _____

Date of adverse reaction (*year/month/day*) _____

Adverse reaction in relation with
- ❑ Whole blood
- ❑ Red blood cells
- ❑ Platelets
- ❑ Plasma
- ❑ Other (*specify*)

Type of adverse reaction(s)
- ❑ Immunological haemolysis due to ABO incompatibility
- ❑ Immunological haemolysis due to other allo-antibody
- ❑ Non-immunological haemolysis
- ❑ Anaphylaxis/hypersensitivity
- ❑ Transfusion-associated circulatory overload (TACO)
- ❑ Transfusion-related acute lung injury (TRALI)
- ❑ Transfusion-transmitted bacterial infection
- ❑ Transfusion-transmitted viral infection (HBV)
- ❑ Transfusion-transmitted viral infection (HCV)
- ❑ Transfusion-transmitted viral infection (HIV-1/2)
- ❑ Transfusion-transmitted viral infection, other (*specify*)
- ❑ Transfusion-transmitted parasitical infection (malaria)
- ❑ Transfusion-transmitted parasitical infection, other (*specify*)
- ❑ Post-transfusion purpura (PTP)

❏ Transfusion-associated – graft versus host disease (TA-GVHD)
❏ Other reaction(s) (*specify*)

Imputability level (NA, 0 to 3): _____

Severity level (1 to 4): _____

ANNEX 5. STANDARDIZED TEMPLATE FORM FOR THE NOTIFICATION OF AN ADVERSE REACTION IN A RECIPIENT: PART B, CONFIRMATION AND FINALIZATION OF THE NOTIFICATION BY THE HOSPITAL

(to be used for an individual incident by the hospital to inform the central haemovigilance unit)

Notification of an adverse reaction

Part B: Confirmation and finalization of a notification for an adverse reaction

Reporting establishment _____

Report identification _____

Date of adverse reaction (*year/month/day*) _____

Confirmation date (*year/month/day*) _____

Confirmation of the adverse reaction
- ❏ Yes
- ❏ No

If No, *specify*: _____

Change of type of adverse reaction
- ❏ Yes
- ❏ No

From initial type: _____
To final type: _____
If Yes, *explain*: _____

Change of imputability level
- ❏ Yes
- ❏ No

From initial imputability level (NA, 0 to 3): _____
To final imputability level (NA, 0 to 3): _____
If Yes, *explain*: _____

Change of severity level
- ❏ Yes
- ❏ No

From initial severity level (1 to 4): _____
To final severity level (1 to 4): _____
If Yes, *explain*: _____

Clinical outcome of the recipient (if known)
- ❏ Complete recovery
- ❏ Minor sequelae (*specify*): _____
- ❏ Serious sequelae (*specify*): _____
- ❏ Death (*give details*): _____

ANNEX 6. STANDARDIZED TEMPLATE FORM FOR THE NOTIFICATION OF AN ADVERSE EVENT IN A HOSPITAL: PART A, RAPID NOTIFICATION

(to be used for an individual incident by the hospital to inform the central haemovigilance unit)

Notification of an adverse event

Part A: <u>Rapid</u> notification of an adverse event

Reporting hospital _____

Report identification _____

Reporting date (*year/month/day*) _____

Date of adverse event (*year/month/day*) _____

Adverse event, which (may) affect the safety of patients to be transfused due to a deviation in:	Specification			
	Product defect	Equipment failure	Human error	Other (*specify*)
Medical prescription				
Patient identification				
Blood sampling				
Blood grouping				
Cross-matching				
Storage of blood products				
Issuing of blood products				
Administration of blood products				
Follow-up of the recipient				
Other (*specify*)				

ANNEX 7. STANDARDIZED TEMPLATE FORM FOR THE NOTIFICATION OF AN ADVERSE EVENT IN A HOSPITAL: PART B, CONFIRMATION AND FINALIZATION OF A NOTIFICATION

(to be used for an individual incident by the hospital to inform the central haemovigilance unit)

Notification of an adverse event

Part B: **Confirmation** and **finalization** of a notification of an adverse event in a hospital

Reporting establishment _____

Report identification _____

Confirmation date (*year/month/day*) _____

Date of adverse event (*year/month/day*) _____

Root cause analysis (*give details*) _____

_____

_____

Corrective measures taken (*give details*) _____

_____

_____

Template for reporting on haemovigilance for the blood establishment

ANNEX 8. STANDARDIZED PERIODIC REPORTING TEMPLATE ON COMPLICATIONS OR ADVERSE REACTIONS OBSERVED IN DONORS BY BLOOD ESTABLISHMENTS

(for internal and external purposes; for monthly, trimestrial, semestrial and annual reporting)

Reporting blood establishment _____

Report identification _____

Reporting period
(*from year/month/day to year/month/day*) _____

Total number of donations (all types) _____

Total number of units (of blood products) distributed to hospitals _____

Total number of units (of blood products) discarded _____

Date of publication (*year/month/day*) _____

This table refers to one of the following types of donation (use a separate table for each blood component):
- ❑ Whole blood
- ❑ Platelets
- ❑ Plasma
- ❑ Combined
- ❑ Other (*specify*): _____

Type of donor complication or adverse reaction(s)	Severity level				
	1	2	3	4	All
Vasovagal					
Total number reported					
Rate per 100 000					
Haematoma					
Total number reported					
Rate per 100 000					
Damage to vessel (vein or artery)					
Total number reported					
Rate per 100 000					
Damage to nerve					
Total number reported					
Rate per 100 000					
Specific apheresis complication					
Total number reported					
Rate per 100 000					
▪ allergic reaction (generalized)					
▪ anaphylaxis					
▪ haemolysis					
▪ embolism					
▪ hypotension (induced due to hypovolemia)					
▪ clotting					
▪ citrate intoxication					
Other reaction(s) (*specify*)					
Total number reported					
Rate per 100 000					

ANNEX 9. STANDARDIZED PERIODIC REPORTING TEMPLATE ON ADVERSE EVENTS OCCURRING IN BLOOD ESTABLISHMENTS

(for internal and external purposes; for monthly, trimestrial, semestrial and annual reporting)

Reporting blood establishment _____

Report identification _____

Reporting period
(*from year/month/day to year/month/day*) _____

Total number of donations (all types) _____

Total number of units (of blood products) distributed to hospitals _____

Total number of units (of blood products) discarded _____

Date of publication (*year/month/day*) _____

Adverse event, which may affect quality and safety of blood component due to a deviation in:	Specification			
	Product defect	Equipment failure	Human error	Other (*specify*)
Whole blood collection				
Total number reported				
Rate per 100 000				
Apheresis collection				
Total number reported				
Rate per 100 000				
Testing of donations				
Total number reported				
Rate per 100 000				
Processing				
Total number reported				
Rate per 100 000				
Storage				
Total number reported				
Rate per 100 000				
Distribution				
Total number reported				
Rate per 100 000				
Materials				
Total number reported				
Rate per 100 000				

Adverse event, which may affect quality and safety of blood component due to a deviation in:	Specification			
	Product defect	Equipment failure	Human error	Other (*specify*)
Others (*specify*)				
Total number reported				
Rate per 100 000				

Template for reporting on haemovigilance for the hospital

ANNEX 10. STANDARDIZED ANNUAL REPORTING TEMPLATE ON ADVERSE REACTIONS OBSERVED IN RECIPIENTS BY HOSPITALS (HEALTH CARE INSTITUTIONS)

(to be used for internal and external purposes, inter alia to inform the central haemovigilance unit)

Reporting hospital _____

Report identification _____

Reporting period
(*from year/month/day to year/month/day*) _____

Total number of patients transfused _____

Total number of units (of blood products) received _____

Total number of units (of blood products) transfused _____

Total number of units (of blood products) discarded _____

Date of publication (*year/month/day*) _____

This table refers to (use a separate table for each blood component):

- ❑ Whole blood
- ❑ Red blood cells
- ❑ Platelets
- ❑ Plasma
- ❑ Other (*specify*): _____

Type of adverse reaction(s) in recipients	Severity level				
	1	2	3	4	All
Immunological haemolysis due to ABO incompatibility					
Immunological haemolysis due to other allo-antibody					
Non-immunological haemolysis					
Anaphylaxis/hypersensitivity					
Transfusion-associated circulatory overload (TACO)					
Transfusion-related acute lung injury (TRALI)					
Transfusion-transmitted bacterial infection					
Transfusion-transmitted viral infection (HBV)					
Transfusion-transmitted viral infection (HCV)					
Transfusion-transmitted viral infection (HIV-1/2)					

Type of adverse reaction(s) in recipients	Severity level				
	1	2	3	4	All
Transfusion-transmitted viral infection, other (specify)					
Transfusion-transmitted parasitical infection (malaria)					
Transfusion-transmitted parasitical infection, other (specify)					
Post-transfusion purpura (PTP)					
Transfusion-associated – graft versus host disease (TA-GVHD)					
Other reaction(s) (*specify*)					

N.B.
This report can further be stratified according to Imputability levels (NA, 0 to 3)
Separate or incorporated in the present one

ANNEX 11. STANDARDIZED ANNUAL REPORTING TEMPLATE ON ADVERSE EVENTS OCCURRING IN HOSPITALS (HEALTH CARE INSTITUTIONS)

(to be used for internal and external purposes, inter alia to inform the central haemovigilance unit)

Reporting hospital _____

Report identification _____

Reporting period
(*from year/month/day to year/month/day*) _____

Total number of patients transfused _____

Total number of units (of blood products) received _____

Total number of units (of blood products) transfused _____

Total number of units (of blood products) discarded _____

Date of publication (*year/month/day*) _____

Adverse event, which may affect the safety of patients to be transfused due to a deviation in:	Specification			
	Product defect	Equipment failure	Human error	Other (*specify*)
Medical prescription				
Total number reported				
Rate per 100 000				
Patient identification				
Total number reported				
Rate per 100 000				
Blood sampling				
Total number reported				
Rate per 100 000				
Blood grouping				
Total number reported				
Rate per 100 000				
Cross-matching				
Total number reported				
Rate per 100 000				
Storage of blood products				
Total number reported				
Rate per 100 000				
Issuing of blood products				
Total number reported				
Rate per 100 000				

Adverse event, which may affect the safety of patients to be transfused due to a deviation in:	Specification			
	Product defect	**Equipment failure**	**Human error**	**Other** (*specify*)
Administration of blood products				
Total number reported				
Rate per 100 000				
Follow-up of the recipient				
Total number reported				
Rate per 100 000				
Others (*specify*)				
Total number reported				
Rate per 100 000				